CW00569975

The Definitive Vegetarian Way to Keto Diet

Tasty and Super - Affordable Keto Recipes for Vegetarian Busy People

Skye Webb

Table of contents

Eggplant Salad 6

Corn And Cabbage Soup 8

Okra Soup 10

Carrot Soup 12

Baby Carrots And Coconut Soup 13

Smokey Cheddar Cheese (vegan) 14

Mozzarella Cheese (vegan) 17

Feta Cheese (vegan) 19

Nut Free Nacho Dip (vegan) 21

Black Olive & Thyme Cheese Spread (vegan) 24

Truffle Parmesan Cheese (vegan) 26

Gorgonzola 'Blue' Cheese (vegan) 28

Zucchini & Ricotta Tart 30

Eggplant Noodles with Sesame Tofu 34

Cheesy Crustless Quiche 37

Rutabaga Hash Browns 39

Twice Baked Spaghetti Squash 42

Curry with Bok Choy 44

Zucchini bread 47

Flax Egg (vegan) 50

Simple Marinara Sauce (vegan) 52

Greek Chia Pudding (lacto) 54

Eggfast Muffins (ovo) 56

Crispy Flaxseed Waffles (ovo) 59

Chocolate-Vanilla Almond Milk (vegan) 61

Nutty Protein Shake (vegan) 62

Chia & Coco Shake (vegan) 64

Fat-Rich Protein Espresso (vegan) 66

Raspberry Protein Shake (vegan) 68

Forest Fruit Blaster (vegan) 70

Lemon Mousse 71

Avocado Pudding 72

Almond Butter Brownies 73

Simple Almond Butter Fudge 75

Chocolate Fudge 76

Coconut Peanut Butter Fudge 77

Raspberry Chia Pudding 79

Quick Choco Brownie 80

CHOCO CHIA PUDDING 81

SMOOTH CHOCOLATE MOUSSE 83

SPICY JALAPENO BRUSSELS SPROUTS 84

SAGE PECAN CAULIFLOWER 85

BAKED CAULIFLOWER 88

CABBAGE CUCUMBER SALAD 90

AVOCADO CUCUMBER SOUP 92

BASIL TOMATO SOUP 93

CREAMY CELERY SOUP 95

ZUCCHINI SOUP 97

LIME CREAM 98

CHERRIES STEW 99

AVOCADO AND ALMOND SWEET CREAM 101

MINT RICE PUDDING 102

WALNUTS AND COCONUT CAKE 104

RHUBARB AND BERRIES CREAM 106

RICE PUDDING 107

STRAWBERRY SORBET 109

CRANBERRIES AND AVOCADO PIE 111

Eggplant Salad

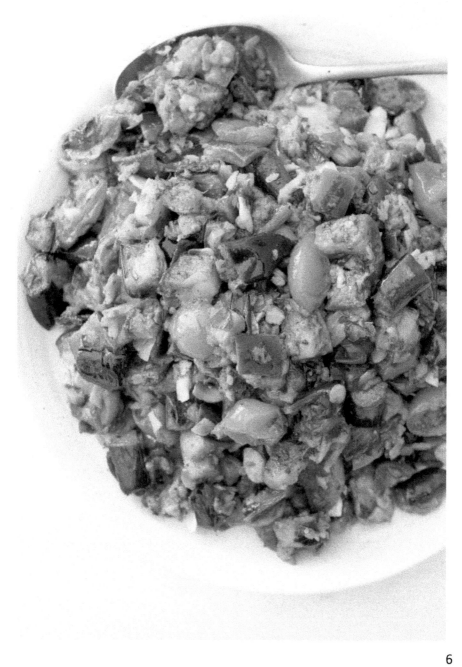

Preparation time: 10 minutes Cooking time: 8 hours Servings: 4

Ingredients:

24 ounces canned tomatoes, chopped 1 red onion, chopped

2 red bell peppers, chopped

1   big eggplant, roughly chopped 1 tablespoon smoked paprika

2   teaspoons cumin, ground

Salt and black pepper to the taste Juice of 1 lemon

1 tablespoons parsley, chopped

Directions:

1.   In your slow cooker, mix tomatoes with onion, bell peppers, eggplant, smoked paprika, cumin, salt, pepper and lemon juice, stir, cover and cook on Low for 8 hours

2.   Add parsley, stir, divide into bowls and serve cold as a dinner salad.

3.   Enjoy!

Nutritions: calories 251, fat 4, fiber 6, carbs 8, protein 3

Corn And Cabbage Soup

Preparation time: 10 minutes Cooking time: 7 hours

Servings: 4

Ingredients:

1   small yellow onion, chopped

1 tablespoon olive oil

2   garlic cloves, minced

1 and ½ cups mushrooms, sliced

3 teaspoons ginger, grated

A pinch of salt and black pepper

2 cups corn kernels

4 cups red cabbage, chopped

4 cups water

1 tablespoon nutritional yeast

2 teaspoons tomato paste

1 teaspoon sesame oil

1 teaspoon coconut aminos

1 teaspoon sriracha sauce

Directions:

1.   In your slow cooker, mix olive oil with onion, garlic, mushrooms, ginger, salt, pepper, corn, cabbage, water, yeast and tomato paste, stir, cover and cook on Low for 7 hours.

2.   Add sriracha sauce and aminos, stir, leave soup aside for a few minutes, ladle into bowls, drizzle sesame oil all over and serve.

3.   Enjoy!

Nutritions: calories 300, fat 4, fiber 4, carbs 10, protein 4

Okra Soup

Preparation time: 10 minutes Cooking time: 5 hours Servings: 6

Ingredients:

1 green bell pepper, chopped

1 small yellow onion, chopped

3 cups veggie stock

3 garlic cloves, minced

16 ounces okra, sliced

2 cup corn

29 ounces canned tomatoes, crushed

1 and ½ teaspoon smoked paprika

1 teaspoon marjoram, dried

1 teaspoon thyme, dried

1   teaspoon oregano, dried

Salt and black pepper to the taste

Directions:

1.   In your slow cooker, mix bell pepper with onion, stock, garlic, okra, corn, tomatoes, smoked paprika, marjoram, thyme, oregano, salt and pepper, stir, cover and cook on High for 5 hours.

2.   Ladle into bowls and serve.

3.   Enjoy!

Nutritions: calories 243, fat 4, fiber 6, carbs 10, protein 3

Carrot Soup

Preparation time: 10 minutes Cooking time: 5 hours Servings: 6

Ingredients:

2   potatoes, cubed

3   pounds carrots, cubed

1 yellow onion, chopped

1-quart veggie stock

Salt and black pepper to the taste

1 teaspoon thyme, dried

3 tablespoons coconut milk

2 teaspoons curry powder

3 tablespoons vegan cheese, crumbled

A handful pistachios, chopped

Directions:

1.   In your slow cooker, mix onion with potatoes, carrots, stock, salt, pepper, thyme and curry powder, stir, cover, cook on High for 1 hour and on Low for 4 hours.

2.   Add coconut milk, stir, blend soup using an immersion blender, ladle soup into bowls, sprinkle vegan cheese and pistachios on top and serve.

3.   Enjoy!

Nutritions: calories 241, fat 4, fiber 7, carbs 10, protein 4

Baby Carrots And Coconut Soup

Preparation time: 10 minutes Cooking time: 7 hours Servings: 6

Ingredients:

1   sweet potato, cubed

2   pounds baby carrots, peeled

2 teaspoons ginger paste

1   yellow onion, chopped

4 cups veggie stock

2   teaspoons curry powder

Salt and black pepper to the taste

14 ounces coconut milk

Directions:

1.   In your slow cooker, mix sweet potato with baby carrots, ginger paste, onion, stock, curry powder, salt and pepper, stir, cover and cook on High for 7 hours.

2.   Add coconut milk, blend soup using an immersion blender, divide soup into bowls and serve.

3.   Enjoy!

Nutritions: calories 100, fat 2, fiber 4, carbs 18, protein 3

Smokey Cheddar Cheese (vegan)

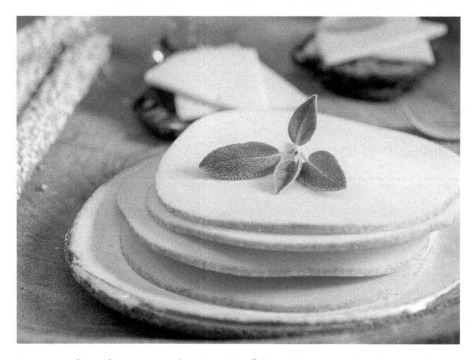

Preparation time: 20 minutes Cooking time: 0 minute Servings: 8

Ingredients:

1 cup raw cashews (unsalted)

1 cup macadamia nuts (unsalted)

4 tsp. tapioca starch

1 cup water

¼ cup fresh lime juice

¼ cup tahini

½ tsp. liquid smoke

¼ cup paprika powder

½ tsp. ground mustard seeds

2 tbsp. onion powder

1 tsp. Himalayan salt

½ tsp. chili powder

1 tbsp. coconut oil

Directions:

1.   Cover the cashews with water in a small bowl and let sit for 4 to 6 hours. Rinse and drain the cashews after soaking. Make sure no water is left.

2.   Mix the tapioca starch with the cup of water in a small saucepan. Heat the pan over medium heat.

3.   Bring the water with tapioca starch to a boil. After 1 minute, take the pan off the heat and set the mixture aside to cool down.

4.   Put all the remaining ingredients—except the coconut oil—in a blender or food processor. Blend until these ingredients are combined into a smooth mixture.

5.   Stir in the tapioca starch with water and blend again until all ingredients have fully incorporated.

6.   Grease a medium-sized bowl with the coconut oil to prevent the cheese from sticking to the edges. Gently pour the mixture into the bowl.

7.   Refrigerate the bowl, uncovered, for about 3 hours until the cheese is firm and ready to enjoy!

8.   Alternatively, store the cheese in an airtight container in the fridge and consume within 6 days. Store for a maximum of 60 days in the freezer and thaw at room temperature.

Nutritions: Calories: 249 kcal, Net Carbs: 6.9g, Fat: 21.7g, Protein: 6.1g, Fiber: 4.3g, Sugar: 2.6g

Mozzarella Cheese (vegan)

Preparation time: 20 minutes Cooking time: 0 minute Servings: 16

Ingredients:

1 cup raw cashews (unsalted)

½ cup macadamia nuts (unsalted)

½ cup pine nuts

½ cup water

½ tbsp. coconut oil

½ tsp. light miso paste

2 tbsp. agar-agar

1 tsp. fresh lime juice

1 tsp. Himalayan salt

Directions:

1.   Cover the cashews with water in a small bowl and let sit for 4 to 6 hours. Rinse and drain the cashews after soaking. Make sure no water is left.

2.   Mix the agar-agar with the ½ cup of water in a small saucepan. Put the pan over medium heat.

3.   Bring the agar-agar mixture to a boil. After 1 minute, take it off the heat and set the mixture aside to cool down.

4.   Put all the other ingredients—except the coconut oil—in a blender or food processor. Blend until everything is well combined.

5.   Add the agar-agar with water and blend again until all ingredients have been fully incorporated.

6.   Grease a medium-sized bowl with the coconut oil to prevent the cheese from sticking to the edges. Gently transfer the cheese mixture into the bowl by using a spatula.

7.   Refrigerate the bowl, uncovered, for about 3 hours until the cheese is firm; then serve and enjoy!

8.   Alternatively, store the cheese in an airtight container in the fridge. Consume within 6 days. Store for a maximum of 60 days in the freezer and thaw at room temperature.

Nutritions: Calories: 101kcal, Net Carbs: 2.1g, Fat: 9.2g, Protein: 2.2g, Fiber: 0.9g, Sugar: 0.9g

Feta Cheese (vegan)

Preparation time: 20 minutes Cooking time: 0 minute Servings: 4

Ingredients:

1 13-oz. block extra firm tofu (drained)

3 cups water

¼ cup apple cider vinegar

2 tbsp. dark miso paste

1 tsp. ground black pepper

2 garlic cloves

1 tbsp. sun dried tomatoes (chopped)

2 tsp. Himalayan salt

Directions:

1.   Cut the tofu into ½-inch cubes and put them into a medium-sized saucepan with 2 cups of water.

2.   Bring the water to a boil over medium-high heat, take the pan off the heat immediately, drain half of the water, and set aside to let it cool down.

3.   Pour the vinegar, miso paste, pepper, salt, and the remaining 1 cup of water into a blender or food processor. Blend until everything is well combined.

4.   Pour the liquid from the blender into an airtight container. Add the garlic cloves, sundried tomatoes, and the tofu (including the water) to the container.

5.   Give the feta cheese a good stir and then store in the fridge or freezer for at least 4 hours before serving.

6.   Serve with low-carb crackers, or, enjoy this delicious feta cheese in a healthy salad!

7.   Alternatively, store the cheese in an airtight container in the fridge and consume within 6 days. Store for a maximum of 30 days in the freezer and thaw at room temperature.

Nutritions: Calories: 101kcal, Carbs: 5.2g, Net Carbs: 3.8g, Fat: 4.9g, Protein: 10.3g, Fiber:1.4g, Sugar: 0.7g

Nut Free Nacho Dip (vegan)

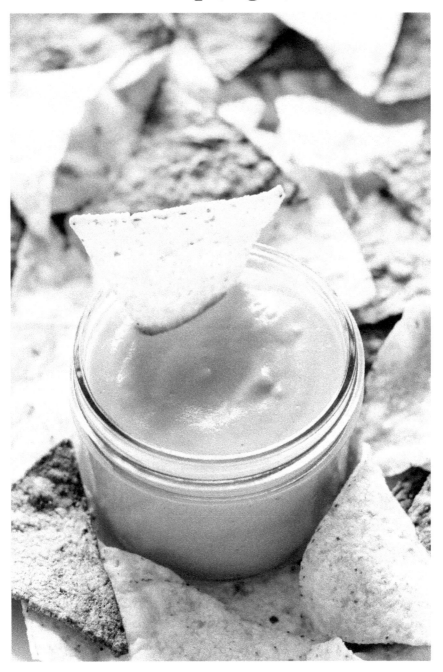

Preparation time: 15 minutes Cooking time: 0 minute Servings: 8

Ingredients:

1   large eggplant (peeled and cubed)

2   medium Hass avocados (peeled, pitted, and halved)

¼ cup MCT oil

2 tsp. nutritional yeast

1 jalapeno pepper

1 red onion (diced)

1 garlic clove (halved)

¼ cup fresh cilantro (chopped)

1 tbsp. paprika powder

1 tsp. cumin seeds

1 tsp. dried oregano

½ tsp. Himalayan salt

Directions:

1.   Slice the jalapeno in half lengthwise; remove the seeds, stem, and placenta, and discard.

2.   Put the jalapeno and all other ingredients in a food processor or blender.

3.   Mix everything into a smooth mixture. Use a spatula to scrape down the sides of the blender to make sure everything gets mixed evenly.

4.   Transfer the dip to an airtight container.

5. Serve, share, and enjoy!

6. Alternatively, store the cheese in an airtight container in the fridge and consume within 2 days.

Nutritions: Calories: 135kcal, Net Carbs: 3.5g, Fat: 12.3g, Protein: 1.8g, Fiber: 5.4g, Sugar: 2.7g

Black Olive & Thyme Cheese Spread (vegan)

Preparation time: 25 minutes Cooking time: 15 minutes Servings: 16

Ingredients:

1 cup macadamia nuts (unsalted)

1 cup pine nuts

1 tsp. thyme (finely chopped)

1 tsp. rosemary (finely chopped)

2 tsp. nutritional yeast

1 tsp. Himalayan salt

10 black olives (pitted, finely chopped)

Directions:

1.   Preheat the oven to 350°F / 175°C, and line a baking sheet with parchment paper.

2.   Put the nuts on a baking sheet, and spread them out so they can roast evenly. Transfer the baking sheet to the oven and roast the nuts for about 8 minutes, until slightly browned.

3.   Take the nuts out of the oven and set aside for about 4 minutes, allowing them to cool down.

4.   Add all ingredients to a blender and process until everything combines into a smooth mixture. Use a spatula to scrape down the sides of the blender container in between blending to make sure everything gets mixed evenly.

5.　　　Serve, share, and enjoy!

6.　　　Alternatively, store the cheese in an airtight container in the fridge and consume within 6 days. Store for a maximum of 60 days in the freezer and thaw at room temperature.

Nutritions: Calories: 118kcal, Net Carbs: 0.7g, Fat: 11.9g, Protein: 2g, Fiber: 1.4g, Sugar: 0.7g

Truffle Parmesan Cheese (vegan)

Preparation time: 30 minutes Cooking time: 0 minute Servings: 8

Ingredients:

1   cup macadamia nuts (unsalted)

1 cup raw cashews (unsalted)

2   garlic cloves

½ tbsp. nutritional yeast

2 tbsp. truffle oil

1 tsp. agar-agar

1 tsp. fresh lime juice

1 tsp. dark miso paste

Directions:

1.   Cover the cashews with water in a small bowl and let sit for 4 to 6 hours. Rinse and drain the cashews after soaking. Make sure no water is left.

2.   Preheat the oven to 350°F / 175°C, and line a baking sheet with parchment paper.

3.   Put the macadamia nuts on a baking sheet and spread them out, so they can roast evenly.

4.   Transfer the baking sheet to the oven and roast the macadamia nuts for about 8 minutes, until slightly browned.

5.   Take the nuts out of the oven and set them aside, allowing them to cool down.

6.   Grease a medium-sized shallow baking dish with ½ tablespoon of truffle oil.

7.   Add the soaked cashews, roasted macadamia nuts, and all the remaining ingredients to a blender or food processor. Blend everything into a crumbly mixture.

8.   Transfer the crumbly parmesan into the baking dish, spread it out evenly, and firmly press it down until it has fused together into an even layer of cheese.

9.   Cover the baking dish with aluminum foil and refrigerate the cheese for 8 hours or until the parmesan is firm.

10.   Serve or store the cheese in an airtight container in the fridge and consume within 6 days. Store for a maximum of 60 days in the freezer and thaw at room temperature.

Nutritions: Calories: 202kcal, Net Carbs: 4.4g, Fat: 18.7g Protein: 4g, Fiber: 1.8g, Sugar: 1.8g

Gorgonzola 'Blue' Cheese (vegan)

Preparation time: 24 hours

Cooking time: 20 minutes Servings: 16

Ingredients:

½ cup macadamia nuts (unsalted)

½ cup pine nuts

1 cup raw cashews (unsalted)

1 capsule acidophilus (probiotic cheese culture)

½ tbsp. MCT oil

¼ cup unsweetened almond milk

1 tsp. ground black pepper

1 tsp. Himalayan salt

1 tsp. spirulina powder

Directions:

1.   Cover the cashews with water in a small bowl and let sit for 4 to 6 hours. Rinse and drain the cashews after soaking. Make sure no water is left.

2.   Preheat the oven to 350°F / 175°C, and line a baking sheet with parchment paper.

3.   Spread the macadamia and pine nuts out on the baking sheet so they can roast evenly.

4.   Put the baking sheet into the oven and roast the nuts for 8 minutes, until they are slightly browned.

5.   Take the nuts out of the oven and allow them to cool down.

6.   Grease a 3-inch cheese mold with the MCT oil and set it aside.

7.   Add all ingredients—except the spirulina—to the blender or food processor. Blend on medium speed into a smooth mixture. Use a spatula to scrape down the sides of the blender to make sure all the ingredients get incorporated.

8.   Transfer the cheese mixture into the greased cheese mold and sprinkle it with the spirulina powder. Use a small teaspoon to create blue marble veins on the cheese, and then cover the mold with parchment paper.

9.   Place the cheese into a dehydrator and dehydrate the cheese at 90°F / 32°C for 24 hours.

10.   Transfer the dehydrated cheese in the covered mold to the fridge. Allow the cheese to refrigerate for 12 hours.

11.   Remove the cheese from the mold to serve in this condition, or, age the cheese in a wine cooler for up to 3 weeks. In case of aging the cheese, rub the outsides of the cheese with fresh sea salt. Refresh the salt every 2 days to prevent any mold. The cheese will develop a blue cheese-like taste, and by aging it, the cheese becomes even more delicious.

12.   If the cheese is not aged, store it in airtight container and consume within 6

days.

13.   Store the aged cheese in an airtight container and consume within 6 days, or for a maximum of 60 days in the freezer and thaw at room temperature.

Nutritions: Calories: 101kcal, Net Carbs: 2g, Fat: 9.3g, Protein: 2.3g, Fiber: 1g, Sugar: 0.9g

Zucchini & Ricotta Tart

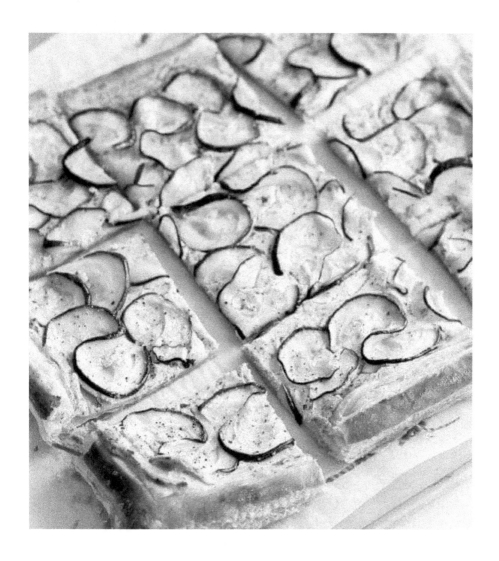

Preparation Time: 25 minutes Cooking Time: about 1 hour
Servings: 8

Ingredients:

For the crust:

1¾ cups almond flour

1 tablespoon coconut flour

½ teaspoon garlic powder

¼ teaspoon salt

¼ cup melted butter

For the filling:

1 medium-large zucchini, thinly sliced cross-wise (use a mandolin if you have one)

½ teaspoon salt

8 ounces ricotta

3 large eggs

¼ cup whipping cream

2 cloves garlic, minced

1 teaspoon fresh dill, minced

Additional salt and pepper to taste

½ cup shredded parmesan

Directions:

To make the crust:

1.   Preheat oven to 325°F.

2.   Lightly spray 9-inch ceramic or glass tart pan with cooking spray.

3.   Combine the almond flour, coconut flour, garlic powder and salt in a large bowl.

4.   Add the butter and stir until dough resembles coarse crumbs.

5.   Press the dough gently into the tart pan, trimming away any excess.

6.   Bake 15 minutes then remove from the oven and let cool.

7.   To make the filling:

8.   While crust is baking, put the zucchini slices into a colander and sprinkle each layer with a little salt. Let sit and drain for 30 minutes.

9.   Place salted zucchini between double layers of paper towels and gently press down to remove any excess water.

10.   Place the ricotta, eggs, whipping cream, garlic, dill, salt and pepper in a bowl and stir well to combine. Add almost all the zucchini slices, reserving about 25-30 for layering on top.

11.   Transfer mixture into cooled crust. Top with the remaining zucchini slices, slightly overlapping.

12.   Sprinkle with parmesan cheese.

13.   Bake 60 to 70 minutes or until center is no longer wobbly and a toothpick

comes out clean.

14.   Cut into slices and serve.

Nutritions: Calories: 302, Total Fats: 25.2g, Carbohydrates: 7.9g, Fiber: 3.1g, Protein: 12.4g

Eggplant Noodles with Sesame Tofu

Preparation Time: 25 minutes Cooking Time: 20-22 minutes Servings: 4

Ingredients:

1 pound block firm tofu

1 cup chopped cilantro

3   tablespoons rice vinegar

4   tablespoons toasted sesame oil

2 cloves garlic, finely minced

1 teaspoon crushed red pepper flakes

2 teaspoons Swerve confectioners

1 whole eggplant

1 tablespoon olive oil

Salt and pepper to taste

¼ cup sesame seeds

¼ cup soy sauce

Directions:

1.   Preheat oven to 200°F.

2.   Remove the block of tofu from packaging. Wrap the tofu in a kitchen towel or paper towels and place a heavy object on top, like a pan or canned goods (alternatively, you can use a tofu press). Let the tofu drain for at least 15 minutes.

3. In a large mixing bowl, add about ¼ cup of cilantro, 3 tablespoons rice vinegar, 2 tablespoons toasted sesame oil, minced garlic, crushed red pepper flakes, and Swerve; whisk together.

4. Peel and julienne the eggplant. You can julienne roughly by hand, or you can use a mandolin with a julienne attachment to cut the eggplant into thin noodles.

5. Add the eggplant into bowl with marinade; toss to coat.

6. Place a skillet over medium-low heat and add olive oil. Once the oil is heated, add the eggplant and cook until it softens. The eggplant will soak up all the liquids, so if you have issues with it sticking to the pan, feel free to add a little more sesame or olive oil. Just be sure to adjust your nutrition tracking.

7. Turn the oven off. Add the remaining cilantro into the eggplant then place the noodles in an oven safe dish. Cover with a lid or foil and place into the oven to keep warm.

8. Pour off fat from skillet then wipe skillet clean with paper towels. Place it back on the stovetop to heat up again.

9. Unwrap the tofu then cut into 8 slices. Spread sesame seeds over a large plate. Press both sides of each tofu slice into the sesame seeds to coat evenly. Transfer to a plate.

10. Pour 2 tablespoons of sesame oil into the skillet.

11. Arrange the tofu slices in a single layer in the skillet and cook on medium-low for about 5 minutes or until they start to crisp. With a spatula, carefully turn them over and cook for about 5 minutes on the other side.

12. Pour ¼ cup of soy sauce into the pan and coat the pieces of tofu. Cook until the tofu slices look browned and caramelized with the soy sauce.

13. To serve, remove the eggplant noodles from the oven, divide them among plates and place the tofu on top.

Nutritions: Calories: 293, Total Fats: 24.4g, Carbohydrates: 12.2g, Fiber: 5.3g, Protein: 11g

Cheesy Crustless Quiche

Preparation Time: 30 minutes Cooking Time: 1 hour

Servings: 6

Ingredients:

6 small Roma tomatoes

½ cup thinly sliced green onion

6 large eggs, beaten

¼ teaspoon Italian Herb Blend

½ teaspoon Spike Seasoning (optional but recommended)

½ cup half and half

1 cup cottage cheese

2 cups shredded Swiss cheese

¼ cup finely grated Parmesan cheese

¼ cup thinly sliced basil

Salt and fresh-ground black pepper to taste

Directions:

1.   Preheat oven to 350°F. Coat a 9-10″ glass or crockery pie dish with non-stick spray.

2.   Cut 3 small Roma tomatoes in half lengthwise and scoop out the seeds. Pat the interior dry with paper towels and then chop the tomatoes.

3.   Break the eggs into a large bowl, add the half and half, Italian Herb Blend, Spike Seasonings, salt and pepper. Whisk until combined.

4.   Stir in the cottage cheese, Swiss cheese, Parmesan cheese, chopped tomatoes, and green onion.

5.   Pour into the prepared pie dish and bake for 30 minutes.

6.   Meanwhile, thinly slice 3 remaining small Roma tomatoes and put on a plate between layers of paper towel. Gently press to help draw out the moisture.

7.   After 30 minutes, remove the quiche from the oven and distribute sliced tomatoes and sliced basil on top of the quiche.

8.   Return to oven and bake an additional 30 minutes or slightly more if the center doesn't seem set enough.

9.   Turn oven to Broil and cook for a minute or two until browned. But keep a close eye on it so the basil does not burn.

10.   Allow the quiche to sit for 5-10 minutes before cutting.

11.   Serve warm or at room temperature.

Nutritions: Calories: 301, Total Fats: 20g, Carbohydrates: 8g, Fiber: 1g, Protein: 23g, Sugar: 4g

Rutabaga Hash Browns

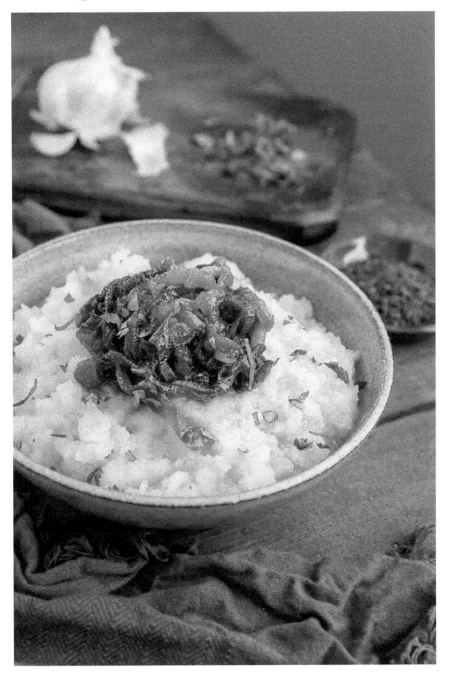

Preparation Time: 20 minutes Cooking Time: 10 minutes Servings: 6

Ingredients:

1 large rutabaga (about 1 pound)

¼ cup finely grated Parmesan cheese

1½ teaspoons dried minced onion

½ teaspoon sea salt

¼ teaspoon black pepper

3 tablespoons avocado oil (or your preferred high-heat tolerant oil)

Directions:

1.   Peel the outer skin from the rutabaga. Chop into about 8 equal pieces.

2.   Bring a medium pot of salted water to a boil. Add peeled & chopped rutabaga and cook over medium- high heat for 10 minutes.

3.   Place the rutabaga pieces in a colander or strainer and rinse them under cold running water then pat dry with a few paper towels.

4.   Shred the rutabaga with either a grater or a food processor equipped with a shredding blade.

5.   Add Parmesan cheese and minced onion to shredded rutabaga, season with salt and pepper, and mix to combine.

6.   Place a large frying pan over medium-low heat and add about 1 tablespoon of oil. Once the oil is heated, add shredded

rutabaga, and cook, working in batches, until crisp and golden brown on one side, 3 to 4 minutes. If desired, gently press the layer down with a spatula. Then use a spatula to flip the rutabaga. Continue to cook until they are golden brown on the bottom, about 3 minutes.

7.   Serve immediately.

Nutritions: Calories: 114, Total Fats: 8g, Carbohydrates: 7g, Fiber: 2g, Protein: 3g

Twice Baked Spaghetti Squash

Preparation Time: 15 minutes Cooking Time: 55 minutes Servings: 6

Ingredients:

2pounds spaghetti squash

1 tablespoon olive oil

¾ cup pecorino romano cheese, shredded (or parmesan)

1 cup mozzarella cheese, shredded

1   teaspoon onion powder

1 tablespoon butter

2   tablespoons fresh thyme leaves

3 cloves garlic, minced

½ teaspoon salt

¼ teaspoon pepper

Directions:

1.   Preheat oven to 400°F.

2.   Use a fork to poke a few holes around the spaghetti squash. Put in the microwave and cook for a minute to soften a bit.

3.   On a cutting board, cut off the end of squash, then cut in half lengthwise. Use a spoon to scrape the pulp and seeds. Rub inside surface with olive oil.

4.   Place each piece of squash, cut side down, onto the baking sheet.

5.   Bake 40-50 minutes or until it has become fork tender.

6.   Let cool for a bit and then use a fork to remove all the strands of spaghetti squash into a mixing bowl.

7.   Put pecorino romano cheese and mozzarella cheese into small dish then add HALF the cheese mixture to the bowl with squash. Add butter, minced garlic, onion powder, fresh thyme, salt and pepper. Using a fork, mash and mix thoroughly to combine everything with the squash flesh.

8.   Spoon this squash mixture back into the skins on a baking sheet pan.

9.   Sprinkle tops with the rest of the cheese mixture and return to oven. Broil 5-6 minutes or until the cheese is melted and starting to brown.

10.   Serve hot.

Nutritions: Calories: 173, Total Fats: 12g, Carbohydrates: 10g, Fiber: 2g

Curry with Bok Choy

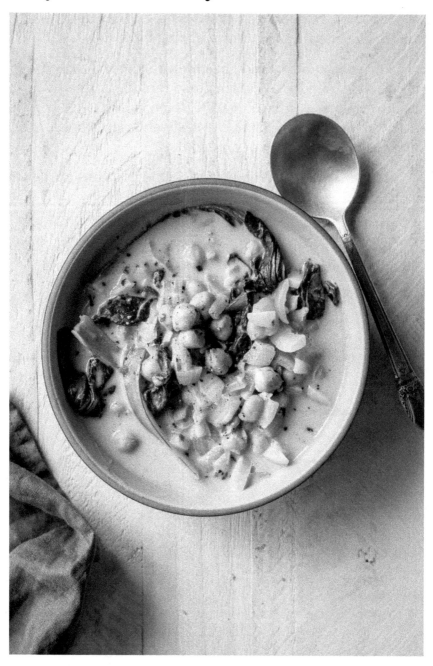

Preparation Time: 15 minutes Cooking Time: 15 minutes Servings: 3

Ingredients:

2 tablespoons extra virgin coconut oil or olive oil

1 small onion, peeled, finely diced

2 cloves garlic, peeled, finely chopped

1 tablespoon curry powder

1   tablespoon fresh grated ginger

½ teaspoon ground turmeric

½ teaspoon ground fenugreek

2   bok choy, washed, feet removed, roughly chopped (14 oz.)
14 oz. unsweetened coconut milk

½ cup vegetable stock

For serving:

Lemon juice

Fresh coriander

Chili flake

Directions:

1.   Place a large skillet over medium heat and add oil. Once the oil is heated, add onions and garlic and cook 1-2 minutes or until golden brown, taking care not to burn them.

2.   Add curry powder, grated ginger, turmeric and fenugreek. Stir fry 30 seconds to1 minute until fragrant.

3.   Stir in bok choy then cover, turn the heat down to medium-low, and cook 3-4 minutes.

4.   Increase the heat to medium-high, uncover and cook 3 - 4 minutes to evaporate the vegetable juice slightly.

5.   Pour in coconut milk and vegetable stock; cook an additional 10 minutes until a thick liquid reduces.

6.   Place curry in a serving bowl. Drizzle with lemon juice. Sprinkle with freshly chopped coriander and chili flakes.

Nutritions: Calories: 200, Total Fats: 15.3g, Carbohydrates: 13.4g, Fiber: 4.8g, Protein: 4.7g, Sugar: 5.2

Zucchini bread

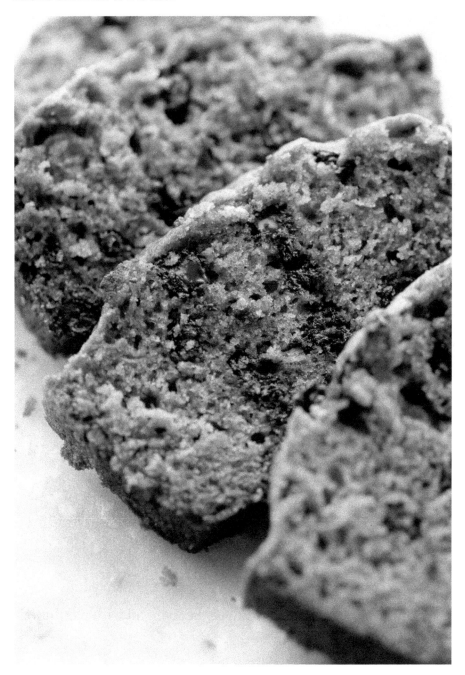

Preparation Time: 20 minutes Cooking Time: 50 minutes Servings: 12

Ingredients:

For the Loaf:

2 cups almond flour

2 teaspoons baking powder

½ teaspoon xanthan gum

¼ teaspoon salt

½ cup coconut oil, melted

¾ cup Swerve granular

3 large eggs

1   teaspoon vanilla extract

2   tablespoons fresh lemon juice

1 tablespoon lemon zest

1 cup zucchini shredded, drained

For the Glaze:

⅓ cup Swerve confectioners 4 tablespoons lemon juice

Directions:

1.   Preheat oven to 325°F. Cover the loaf pan with parchment paper.

2.   Combine flour, salt, baking powder, and xanthan gum in a bowl. Mix well.

3.   In a separate medium bowl, whisk together oil, Swerve granular, eggs, vanilla, and lemon juice.

4.   Add the wet ingredients to the dry ingredients and mix until just combined.

5.   Fold the zucchini and lemon zest into the batter.

6.   Pour the batter into the prepared loaf pan and bake until a toothpick inserted into the middle comes out clean, about 50 minutes. If you find your zucchini bread is browning too quickly, you can cover the pan with foil.

7.   Remove from the oven and let the bread cool in the pan for 10 minutes. Carefully remove the bread from the pan and cool completely on a wire rack.

8.   Whisk together Swerve confectioners and lemon juice. Drizzle loaf with glaze.

9.   Slice and serve.

Nutritions: Calories: 143, Total Fats: 13g, Carbohydrates: 2g, Fiber: 1g, Protein: 2g

Flax Egg (vegan)

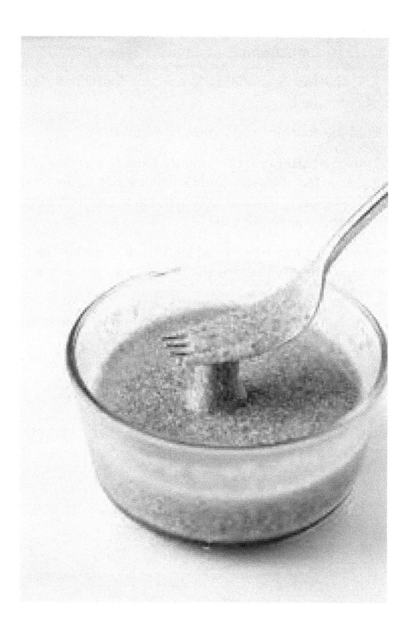

Preparation Time: 12 minutes Cooking Time: 0 minute Servings: 1

Ingredients:

1 tbsp. ground flaxseed

2-3 tbsp. lukewarm water

Directions:

1.   Mix the ground flaxseed and water in a small bowl by using a spoon.

2.   Cover the mixture and let it sit for 10 minutes.

3.   Use the flax egg immediately, or, store it in an airtight container in the fridge and consume within 5 days.

Nutritions: Calories: 37kcal, Net Carbs: 0.2g, Fat: 2.7g, Protein: 1.1g, Fiber: 1.9g, Sugar: 0g

Simple Marinara Sauce (vegan)

Preparation Time: 10 minutes Cooking Time: 10 minutes Servings: 8

Ingredients:

3 tbsp. olive oil

1   14-oz. can peeled tomatoes (no sugar added)

⅓ cup red onion (diced)

2 garlic cloves (minced)

2   tbsp. oregano (fresh and chopped, or 1 tbsp. dried)

½ tsp. cayenne pepper

Optional: 1 tbsp. sunflower seed butter (use grass-fed butter for a lacto sauce)

Directions:

1.   Heat the olive oil in a medium-sized skillet over medium heat.

2.   Add the onions, garlic, salt, and cayenne pepper. Sauté the onions until translucent while stirring the ingredients.

3.   Add the peeled tomatoes and more salt and pepper to taste.

4.   Stir the ingredients, cover the skillet, and allow the sauce to softly cook for 10 minutes.

5.   Add the oregano, and if desired, stir in the optional butter.

6.   Take the skillet off the heat. The sauce is now ready to be used in a recipe!

7.   Alternatively, store the sauce in an airtight container in the fridge and consume within 3 days. Store for a maximum of 30 days in the freezer and thaw at room temperature.

Nutritions: Calories: 23kcal, Net Carbs: 2.8g, Fat: 1.1g, Protein: 0.7g, Fiber: 0.9g, Sugar: 0.1g

Greek Chia Pudding (lacto)

Preparation Time: 20 minutes Cooking Time: 0 minute Servings: 3

Ingredients:

1 cup full-fat Greek yogurt

½ cup full-fat coconut milk

½ scoop organic soy protein powder (vanilla or chocolate flavor)

5 tbsp. chia seeds

4-6 drops stevia sweetener (or alternatively, use low-carb maple syrup)

¼ cup raspberries

¼ cup pecans (crushed)

Optional: 1-2 tbsp. water

Directions:

1.   In a medium-sized bowl, mix the yogurt with the coconut milk.

2.   Stir in the protein powder and chia seeds until the protein powder is fully incorporated. Add some water if necessary.

3.   Allow the pudding to sit for 2 minutes; then add the stevia sweetener and give the yogurt another stir.

4.   Refrigerate the pudding overnight (or for at least 8 hours). This will guarantee a perfect pudding.

5.   Top the pudding with the raspberries and crushed pecans; serve and enjoy!

6. Alternatively, store the pudding in an airtight container and keep it in the fridge and consume within 4 days. Or, you can freeze the pudding for a maximum of 30 days and thaw at room temperature.

Nutritions: Calories: 318kcal, Net Carbs: 6.5g, Fat: 26.6g, Protein: 11.9g, Fiber: 7.4g, Sugar: 4g

Eggfast Muffins (ovo)

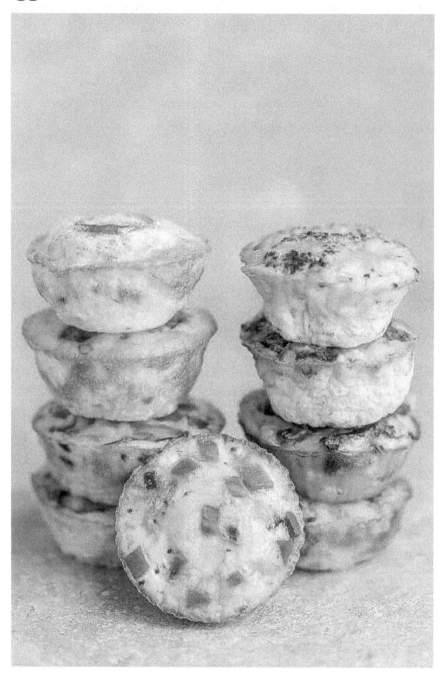

Preparation Time: 15 minutes Cooking Time: 25 minutes
Servings: 9

Ingredients:

9 large organic eggs

1 cup mushrooms (sliced)

½ cup scallions (finely chopped)

1   cup broccoli florets (stems removed)

4 tbsp. sugar-free sweet hot sauce

Sea salt and pepper to taste

¼ cup fresh parsley (chopped)

Directions:

1.   Preheat oven to 375°F / 190°C, and line a 9-cup muffin tray
with muffin liners.

2.   Take a large bowl, crack the eggs in it, and whisk while
adding salt and pepper to taste.

3.   Add all the remaining ingredients to the bowl and stir
thoroughly.

4.   Fill each muffin liner with the egg mixture. Repeat this for
all 9 muffins.

5.   Transfer the tray to the oven and bake for about 30
minutes, or until the muffins have risen and browned on top.

6.   Take the tray out of the oven, and let the muffins cool down
for about 2 minutes; serve and enjoy.

7.   Alternatively, store the muffins in an airtight container in the fridge, and consume within 3 days. Store for a maximum of 30 days in the freezer and thaw at room temperature. Use a microwave, toaster oven, or pan to reheat the omelet.

Nutritions: Calories: 76kcal, Net Carbs: 1.1g, Fat: 4.9g,Protein: 6.9g. Fiber: 0.4g, Sugar: 0.6g

Crispy Flaxseed Waffles (ovo)

Preparation Time: 15 minutes Cooking Time: 20 minutes Servings: 8

Ingredients:

2 cups golden flaxseed (if available, use golden flaxseed meal) 1 tbsp. baking powder

5 large organic eggs (for vegan waffles, replace with 5 flax eggs)

½ cup water (slightly more if necessary)

⅓ cup extra virgin olive oil

1 tbsp. ground cinnamon

1 tbsp. pure vanilla extract

6-12 drops stevia sweetener (or more depending on desired sweetness)

Pinch of salt

Optional: ¼ cup toasted coconut flakes

Directions:

1. Preheat a waffle maker. If you don't have a waffle maker, heat a medium-sized skillet over medium- high heat for crispy flaxseed pancakes. Grease the waffle maker or skillet with a pinch of olive oil.

2. Take a medium-sized bowl and combine the flaxseed (or flaxseed meal) with the baking powder, eggs, water, remaining olive oil, and a pinch of salt. Incorporate all ingredients by using a whisk and allow the mixture to sit for 5 minutes.

3.   Transfer the mixture to a blender or food processor and blend until foamy.

4.   Pour the mixture back into the bowl and allow it to sit for another 3 minutes.

5.   Add the remaining dry ingredients—except the optional toasted coconut flakes—and incorporate everything by using a whisk.

6.   Scoop ¼ of the mixture into the waffle maker or skillet. Cook until a firm waffle or pancake has formed. When using a skillet, carefully flip the pancake.

7.   Repeat this process for the 3 remaining parts of the batter.

8.   Serve the waffles (or pancakes) with the optional toasted coconut flakes and enjoy!

9.   Alternatively, store the waffles in an airtight container, keep them in the fridge, and consume within 3 days. Store for a maximum of 30 days in the freezer and thaw at room temperature.

Nutritions: Calories: 204kcal, Net Carbs: 1.5g, Fat: 18g, Protein: 8g, Fiber: 5.9g, Sugar: 0.3g

Chocolate-Vanilla Almond Milk (vegan)

Preparation Time: 5 minutes Cooking Time: 0 minute Servings: 1

Ingredients:

2   tbsp. coconut oil

1½ cups unsweetened almond milk

½ vanilla stick (crushed)

1   scoop organic soy protein powder (chocolate flavor)

4-6 drops stevia sweetener

Optional: ½ tsp. cinnamon Optional: 1-2 ice cubes

Directions:

1.   Add all the listed ingredients to a blender—except the ice—but including the optional cinnamon if desired.

2.   Blend the ingredients for 1 minute; then if desired, add the optional ice cubes and blend for another 30 seconds.

3.   Transfer the milk to a large cup or shaker, top with some additional cinnamon, serve, and enjoy!

4.   Alternatively, store the smoothie in an airtight container or a mason jar, keep it in the fridge, and consume within 3 days. Store for a maximum of 30 days in the freezer and thaw at room temperature.

Nutritions: Calories: 422kcal, Net Carbs: 1.3g, Fat: 34.8g, Protein: 25.5g, Fiber: 2.7g, Sugar: 0.8g

Nutty Protein Shake (vegan)

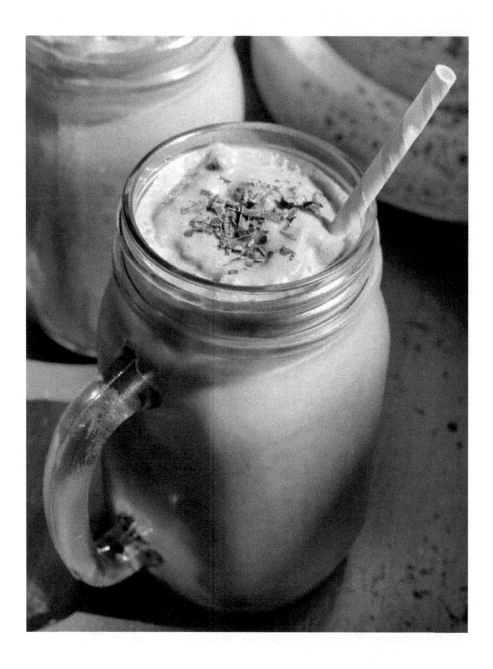

Preparation Time: 5 minutes Cooking Time: 0 minute Servings: 1

Ingredients:

2   tbsp. coconut oil

2 cups unsweetened almond milk

2 tbsp. peanut butter

1 scoop organic soy protein powder (chocolate flavor)

2-4 ice cubes

4-6 drops stevia sweetener

Optional: 1 tsp. vegan creamer

Optional: 1 tsp. cocoa powder

Directions:

1.   Add all the above listed ingredients—except the optional ingredients—to a blender, and blend for 2 minutes.

2.   Transfer the shake to a large cup or shaker. If desired, top the shake with the optional vegan creamer and/or cocoa powder.

3.   Stir before serving, and enjoy!

4.   Alternatively, store the smoothie in an airtight container or a mason jar, keep it in the fridge, and consume within 3 days. Store for a maximum of 30 days in the freezer and thaw at room temperature.

Nutritions: Calories: 618kcal, Net Carbs: 4.4g, Fat: 51.3g, Protein: 34g, Fiber: 4.9g, Sugar: 3g

Chia & Coco Shake (vegan)

Preparation Time: 5 minutes Cooking Time: 0 minute Servings: 2

Ingredients:

1 tbsp. chia seeds

6 tbsp. water

1   cup full-fat coconut milk

2   tbsp. peanut butter (see recipe)

1 tbsp. MCT oil (or coconut oil)

1 scoop organic soy protein powder (chocolate flavor)

Pinch of Himalayan salt

2-4 ice cubes or ½ cup of water

Directions:

1.   Mix the chia seeds and 6 tablespoons of water in a small bowl; let sit for at least 30 minutes.

2.   Transfer the soaked chia seeds and all other listed ingredients to a blender and blend for 2 minutes.

3.   Transfer the shake to a large cup or shaker, serve, and enjoy!

4.   Alternatively, store the smoothie in an airtight container or a mason jar, keep it in the fridge, and consume within 3 days. Store for a maximum of 30 days in the freezer and thaw at room temperature.

Nutritions: Calories: 509kcal, Net Carbs: 5.4g, Fat: 44.55g, Protein: 20.3g, Fiber: 7.45g, Sugar: 3.5g

Fat-Rich Protein Espresso (vegan)

Preparation Time: 5 minutes Cooking Time: 0 minute Servings: 1

Ingredients:

1   cup espresso (freshly brewed)

2   tbsp. coconut butter (or alternatively, use coconut oil)

1 scoop organic soy protein (chocolate flavor)

½ vanilla stick

4 ice cubes or ½ cup boiled water

Optional: 1 tbsp. cacao powder

Optional: ½ tsp. cinnamon

2 tbsp. coconut cream

Directions:

1.   Make sure to use fresh, hot espresso.

2.   Add all the listed ingredients to a heat-safe blender, including the ice or boiled water and optional ingredients (if desired). Use ice to make iced espresso, or hot water for a warm treat.

3.   Blend the ingredients for 1 minute and transfer to a large coffee cup.

4.   Top the coffee with the coconut cream, stir, serve and enjoy!

5.   Alternatively, store the smoothie in an airtight container or a mason jar, keep it in the fridge, and consume within 3 days.

Store for a maximum of 30 days in the freezer and thaw at room temperature.

Nutritions: Calories: 441kcal, Net Carbs: 5.6g, Fat: 34.8g, Protein: 25.4g, Fiber: 6.9g, Sugar: 2.8g

Raspberry Protein Shake (vegan)

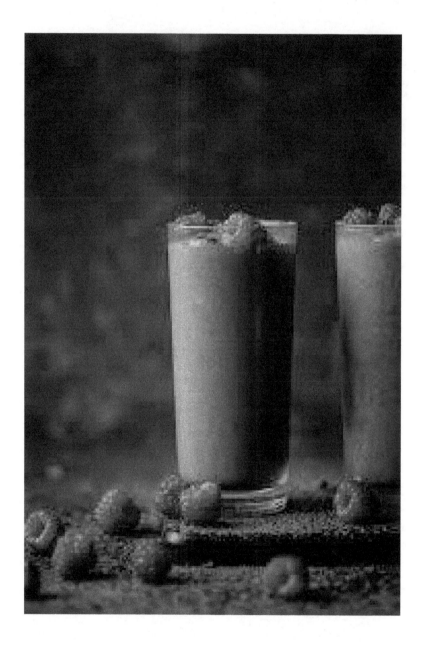

Preparation Time: 5 minutes Cooking Time: 0 minute Servings: 2

Ingredients:

1 cup full-fat coconut milk (or alternatively, use almond milk)

Optional: ¼ cup coconut cream

1   scoop organic soy protein (chocolate or vanilla flavor)

½ cup raspberries (fresh or frozen)

1 tbsp. low-carb maple syrup

Optional: 2-4 ice cubes

Directions:

1.   Add all the ingredients to a blender, including the optional coconut cream and ice cubes if desired, and blend for 1 minute.

2.   Transfer the shake to a large cup or shaker, and enjoy!

3.   Alternatively, store the smoothie in an airtight container or a mason jar, keep it in the fridge, and consume within 2 days. Store for a maximum of 30 days in the freezer and thaw at room temperature.

Nutritions: Calories: 311kcal, Net carbs: 4.6g, Fat: 25.7g, Protein: 14.65g, Fiber: 3.5g, Sugar: 3.35g

Forest Fruit Blaster (vegan)

Preparation Time: 5 minutes Cooking Time: 0 minute Servings: 4

Ingredients:

¼ cup mixed berries (fresh or frozen)

½ kiwi (peeled)

2   cups full-fat coconut milk

2 scoops organic soy protein (vanilla flavor)

½ cup water

Optional: 2 ice cubes

Directions:

1.   Add all the ingredients to a blender, including the optional ice if desired, and blend for 1 minute.

2.   Transfer the shake to a large cup or shaker, and enjoy!

3.   Alternatively, store the smoothie in an airtight container or a mason jar, keep it in the fridge, and consume within 2 days. Store for a maximum of 30 days in the freezer and thaw at room temperature.

Nutritions: Calories: 275kcal, Fat:24.8g, Protein: 8.5g, Net carbs: 4g, Fiber: 1.9g, Sugar: 3.4g

Lemon Mousse

Preparation Time: 10 minutes Cooking Time: 0 minute Servings: 2

Ingredients:

14 oz coconut milk

12 drops liquid stevia

1/2 tsp lemon extract

1/4 tsp turmeric

Directions:

1.   Place coconut milk can in the refrigerator for overnight. Scoop out thick cream into a mixing bowl.

2.   Add remaining ingredients to the bowl and whip using a hand mixer until smooth.

3.   Transfer mousse mixture to a zip-lock bag and pipe into small serving glasses. Place in refrigerator.

4.   Serve chilled and enjoy.

Nutritions: Calories 444, Fat 45.7g, Carbohydrates 10g, Sugar 6g, Protein 4.4g, Cholesterol 0mg

Avocado Pudding

Preparation Time: 10 minutes Cooking Time: 0 minute Servings: 8

Ingredients:

2 ripe avocados, peeled, pitted and cut into pieces

1 tbsp fresh lime juice

14 oz can coconut milk

80 drops of liquid stevia

2 tsp vanilla extract

Directions:

1.   Add all ingredients into the blender and blend until smooth.

2.   Serve and enjoy.

Nutritions: Calories 317, Fat 30.1g. Carbohydrates 9.3g, Sugar 0.4g, Protein 3.4g, Cholesterol 0mg

Almond Butter Brownies

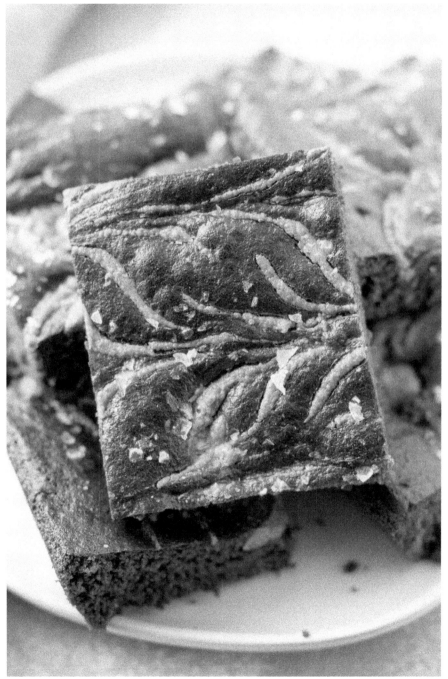

Preparation Time: 15 minutes Cooking Time: 15 minutes

Servings: 4

Ingredients:

1 scoop protein powder

2 tbsp cocoa powder

1/2 cup almond butter, melted

1 cup bananas, overripe

Directions:

1.   Preheat the oven to 350 F/ 176 C.

2.   Spray brownie tray with cooking spray.

3.   Add all ingredients into the blender and blend until smooth.

4.   Pour batter into the prepared dish and bake in preheated oven for 20 minutes.

5.   Serve and enjoy.

Nutritions: Calories 82, Fat 2.1g, Carbohydrates 11.4g, Protein 6.9g, Sugars 5g, Cholesterol 16mg

Simple Almond Butter Fudge

Preparation Time: 15 minutes Cooking Time: 0 minute Servings: 8

Ingredients:

1/2 cup almond butter

15 drops liquid stevia

2 1/2 tbsp coconut oil

Directions:

1.   Combine together almond butter and coconut oil in a saucepan. Gently warm until melted.

2.   Add stevia and stir well.

3.   Pour mixture into the candy container and place in refrigerator until set.

4.   Serve and enjoy.

Nutritions: Calories 43, Fat 4.8g, Carbohydrates 0.2g, Protein 0.2g, Sugars 0g, Cholesterol 0mg

Chocolate Fudge

Preparation Time: 10 minutes Cooking Time: 0 minute Servings: 12

Ingredients:

4 oz unsweetened dark chocolate

3/4 cup coconut butter

15 drops liquid stevia

1 tsp vanilla extract

Directions:

1.   Melt coconut butter and dark chocolate.

2.   Add ingredients to the large bowl and combine well.

3.   Pour mixture into a silicone loaf pan and place in refrigerator until set.

4.   Cut into pieces and serve.

Nutritions: Calories 157, Fat 14.1g, Carbohydrates 6.1g, Sugar 1g, Protein 2.3g, Cholesterol 0mg

Coconut Peanut Butter Fudge

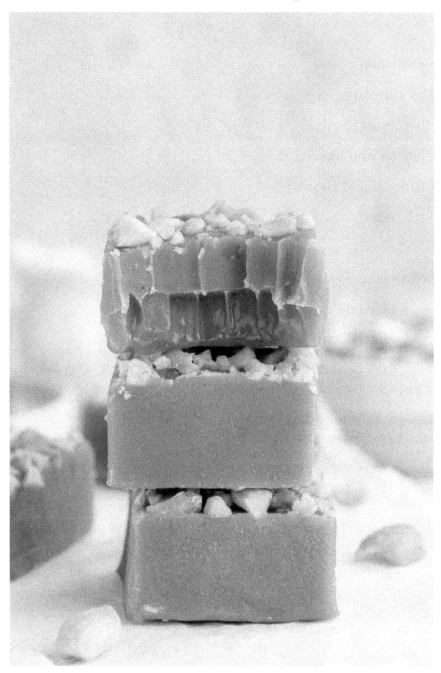

Preparation Time: 10 minutes Cooking Time: 0 minute Servings: 12

Ingredients:

12 oz smooth peanut butter

3 tbsp coconut oil

4 tbsp coconut cream

15 drops liquid stevia

Pinch of salt

Directions:

1.   Line baking tray with parchment paper.

2.   Melt coconut oil in a saucepan over low heat.

3.   Add peanut butter, coconut cream, stevia, and salt in a saucepan. Stir well.

4.   Pour fudge mixture into the prepared baking tray and place in refrigerator for 1 hour.

5.   Cut into pieces and serve.

Nutritions: Calories 125, Fat 11.3g, Carbohydrates 3.5g Sugar 1.7g, Protein 4.3g, Cholesterol 0mg

Raspberry Chia Pudding

Preparation Time: 3 hours & 10 minutes Cooking Time: 0 minute

Servings: 2

Ingredients:

4 tbsp chia seeds

1 cup coconut milk

1/2 cup raspberries

Directions:

1. Add raspberry and coconut milk in a blender and blend until smooth.

2. Pour mixture into the Mason jar.

3. Add chia seeds in a jar and stir well.

4. Close jar tightly with lid and shake well.

5. Place in refrigerator for 3 hours.

6. Serve chilled and enjoy.

Nutritions: Calories 361, Fat 33.4g, Carbohydrates 13.3g, Sugar 5.4g, Protein 6.2g, Cholesterol 0mg

Quick Choco Brownie

Preparation Time: 10 minutes Cooking Time: 0 minute Servings: 1

Ingredients:

1/4 cup almond milk

1 tbsp cocoa powder

1 scoop chocolate protein powder

1/2 tsp baking powder

Directions:

1.   In a microwave-safe mug blend together baking powder, protein powder, and cocoa.

2.   Add almond milk in a mug and stir well.

3.   Place mug in microwave and microwave for 30 seconds.

4.   Serve and enjoy.

Nutritions: Calories 207, Fat 15.8g, Carbohydrates 9.5g, Sugar 3.1g, Protein 12.4g, Cholesterol 20mg

Choco Chia Pudding

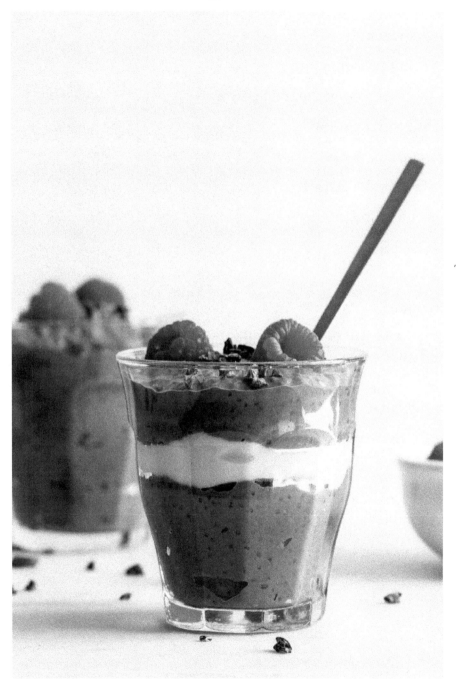

Preparation Time: 10 minutes Cooking Time: 0 minute Servings: 6

Ingredients:

2 1/2 cups coconut milk

2   scoops stevia extract powder

6 tbsp cocoa powder

1/2 cup chia seeds

1/2 tsp vanilla extract

1/8 cup xylitol

1/8 tsp salt

Directions:

1.   Add all ingredients into the blender and blend until smooth.

2.   Pour mixture into the glass container and place in refrigerator.

3.   Serve chilled and enjoy.

Nutritions: Calories 259, Fat 25.4g, Carbohydrates 10.2g, Sugar 3.5g, Protein 3.8g, Cholesterol 0mg

Smooth Chocolate Mousse

Preparation Time: 10 minutes

Cooking Time: 0 minute Servings: 2

Ingredients:

1/2 tsp cinnamon

3   tbsp unsweetened cocoa powder

1 cup creamed coconut milk

10 drops liquid stevia

Directions:

1.   Place coconut milk can in the refrigerator for overnight; it should get thick and the solids separate from water.

2.   Transfer thick part into the large mixing bowl without water.

3.   Add remaining ingredients to the bowl and whip with electric mixer until smooth.

4.   Serve and enjoy.

Nutritions: Calories 296, Fat 29.7g, Carbohydrates 11.5g, Sugar 4.2g, Protein 4.4g, Cholesterol 0mg

Spicy Jalapeno Brussels sprouts

Preparation Time: 5 minutes Cooking Time: 10 minutes Servings: 4

Ingredients:

1 lb Brussels sprouts

1 medium onion, chopped

1 tbsp olive oil

1 jalapeno pepper, seeded and chopped

Pepper

Salt

Directions:

1.   Heat olive oil in a pan over medium heat.

2.   Add onion and jalapeno in the pan and sauté until softened.

3.   Add Brussels sprouts and stir until golden brown, about 10 minutes.

4.   Season with pepper and salt.

5.   Serve and enjoy.

Nutritions: Calories 91, Fat 3.9g, Carbohydrates 13.1g, Sugar 3.7g, Protein 4.2g, Cholesterol 0mg

Sage Pecan Cauliflower

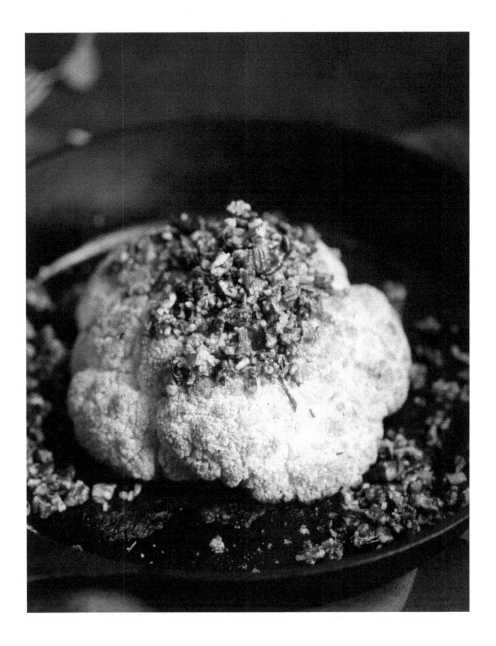

Preparation Time: 10 minutes Cooking Time: 30 minutes Servings: 6

Ingredients:

1   large cauliflower head, cut into florets

1/2 tsp dried thyme

1/2 tsp poultry seasoning

1/4 cup olive oil

2   garlic clove, minced

1/4 cup pecans, chopped

2 tbsp parsley, chopped

1/2 tsp ground sage

1/4 cup celery, chopped

1   onion, sliced

1/4 tsp black pepper

1 tsp sea salt

Directions:

1.   Preheat the oven to 450 F/ 232 C.

2.   Spray a baking tray with cooking spray and set aside.

3.   In a large bowl, mix together cauliflower, thyme, poultry seasoning, olive oil, garlic, celery, sage, onions, pepper, and salt.

4.   Spread mixture on a baking tray and roast in preheated oven for 15 minutes.

5. Add pecans and parsley and stir well. Roast for 10-15 minutes more.

6. Serve and enjoy.

Nutritions: Calories 118, Fat 8.6g, Carbohydrates 9.9g, Sugar 4.2g, Protein 3.1g, Cholesterol 0mg

Baked Cauliflower

Preparation Time: 15 minutes Cooking Time: 40 minutes Servings: 2

Ingredients:

1/2 cauliflower head, cut into florets

2 tbsp olive oil

For seasoning:

1/2 tsp garlic powder

1/2 tsp ground cumin

1/2 tsp black pepper

1/2 tsp white pepper

1 tsp onion powder

1/4 tsp dried oregano

1/4 tsp dried basil

1/4 tsp dried thyme

1   tbsp ground cayenne pepper

2 tbsp ground paprika

2   tsp salt

Directions:

1.   Preheat the oven to 400 F/ 200 C.

2.   Spray a baking tray with cooking spray and set aside.

3.   In a large bowl, mix together all seasoning ingredients.

4.   Add oil and stir well. Add cauliflower to the bowl seasoning mixture and stir well to coat.

5.   Spread the cauliflower florets on a baking tray and bake in preheated oven for 45 minutes.

6.   Serve and enjoy.

Nutritions: Calories 177, Fat 15.6g, Carbohydrates 11.5g, Sugar 3.2g, Protein 3.1g, Cholesterol 0mg

Cabbage Cucumber Salad

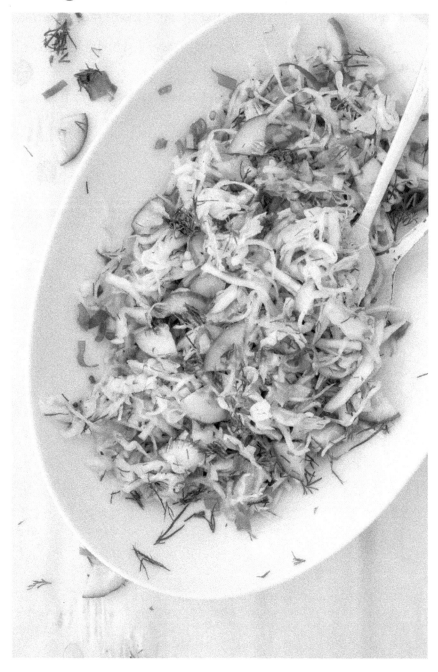

Preparation Time: 20 minutes Cooking Time: 0 minute

Servings: 8

Ingredients:

1/2 cabbage head, chopped

2 cucumbers, sliced

2 tbsp green onion, chopped

2   tbsp fresh dill, chopped

3 tbsp olive oil

1/2 lemon juice

Pepper

Salt

Directions:

1.   Add cabbage to the large bowl. Season with 1 teaspoon of salt mix well and set aside.

2.   Add cucumbers, green onions, and fresh dill. Mix well.

3.   Add lemon juice, pepper, olive oil, and salt. Mix well.

4.   Place salad bowl in refrigerator for 2 hours.

5.   Serve chilled and enjoy.

Nutritions: Calories 71, Fat 5.4g, Carbohydrates 5.9g, Sugar 2.8g, Protein 1.3g, Cholesterol 0mg

Avocado Cucumber Soup

Preparation Time: 40 minutes Cooking Time: 0 minute

Servings: 3

Ingredients:

1 large cucumber, peeled and sliced

¾ cup water

¼ cup lemon juice

2 garlic cloves

6 green onion

2 avocados, pitted

½ tsp black pepper

½ tsp pink salt

Directions:

1.   Add all ingredients into the blender and blend until smooth and creamy.

2.   Place in refrigerator for 30 minutes.

3.   Stir well and serve chilled.

Nutritions: Calories 73, Fat 3.7g, Carbohydrates 9.2g, Sugar 2.8g, Protein 2.2g, Cholesterol 0mg

Basil Tomato Soup

Preparation Time: 5 minutes Cooking Time: 15 minutes Servings: 6

Ingredients:

28 oz can tomatoes

¼ cup basil pesto

¼ tsp dried basil leaves

1 tsp apple cider vinegar

2 tbsp erythritol

¼ tsp garlic powder

½ tsp onion powder

2 cups water

1 ½ tsp kosher salt

Directions:

1.   Add tomatoes, garlic powder, onion powder, water, and salt in a saucepan.

2.   Bring to boil over medium heat. Reduce heat and simmer for 2 minutes.

3.   Remove saucepan from heat and puree the soup using a blender until smooth.

4.   Stir in pesto, dried basil, vinegar, and erythritol.

5.   Stir well and serve warm.

Nutritions: Calories 30, Fat 0g, Carbohydrates 12.1g, Sugar 9.6g, Protein 1.3g, Cholesterol 0mg

Creamy Celery Soup

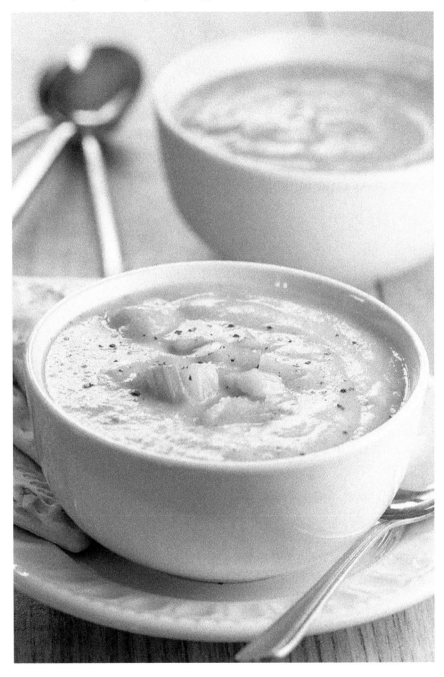

Preparation Time: 15 minutes Cooking Time: 25 minutes Servings: 4

Ingredients:

6 cups celery

½ tsp dill

2 cups water

1   cup coconut milk

1 onion, chopped

Pinch of salt

Directions:

1.   Add all ingredients into the instant pot and stir well.

2.   Cover instant pot with lid and select soup setting.

3.   Release pressure using quick release method than open the lid.

4.   Puree the soup using an immersion blender until smooth and creamy.

5.   Stir well and serve warm.

Nutritions: Calories 174, Fat 14.6g, Carbohydrates 10.5g, Sugar 5.2g, Protein 2.8g, Cholesterol 0mg

Zucchini Soup

Preparation Time: 10 minutes Cooking Time: 10 minutes Servings: 8

Ingredients:

2   ½ lbs zucchini, peeled and sliced

1/3 cup basil leaves

4 cups vegetable stock

4 garlic cloves, chopped

2 tbsp olive oil

1 medium onion, diced

Pepper

Salt

Directions:

1.   Heat olive oil in a pan over medium-low heat.

2.   Add zucchini and onion and sauté until softened. Add garlic and sauté for a minute.

3.   Add vegetable stock and simmer for 15 minutes.

4.   Remove from heat. Stir in basil and puree the soup using a blender until smooth and creamy. Season with pepper and salt.

5.   Stir well and serve.

Nutritions: Calories 62, Fat 4g, Carbohydrates 6.8g, Sugar 3.3g, Protein 2g, Cholesterol 0mg

Lime Cream

Preparation time: 1 hour Cooking time: 0 minutes Servings: 6

Ingredients:

2   tablespoons flaxseed mixed with 3 tablespoons water

1 cup stevia

5 tablespoons avocado oil

1 cup coconut cream

Juice of 1 lime

Zest of 1 lime, grated

Directions:

1.   In a blender, combine the flaxseed mix with the stevia, the oil and the other ingredients, pulse well, divide into cups and keep in the fridge for 1 hour before serving.

Nutrition: calories 200, fat 8.5, fiber 4.5, carbs 8.6, protein 4.5

Cherries Stew

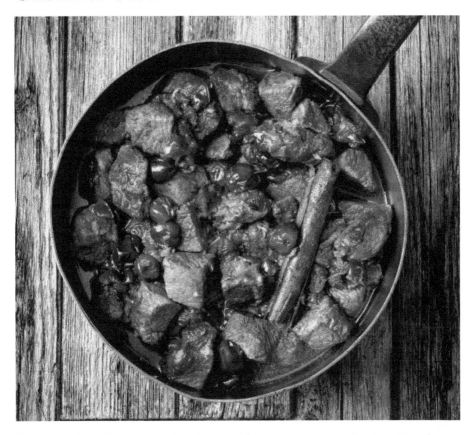

Preparation time: 10 minutes Cooking time: 10 minutes Servings: 4

Ingredients:

2 cups cherries, pitted

 3 tablespoons stevia

2 cups water

1   tablespoon mint, chopped

1 teaspoon vanilla extract

Directions:

1.   In a pan, combine the cherries with the stevia, water and the other ingredients, stir, bring to a simmer and cook over medium-low heat for 10 minutes.

2.   Divide into cups and serve cold.

Nutrition: calories 192, fat 5.4, fiber 3.4, carbs 9.4, protein 4.5

Avocado and Almond Sweet Cream

Preparation time: 20 minutes Cooking time: 0 minutes Servings: 6

Ingredients:

2   avocados, peeled, pitted and mashed

1 cup coconut cream

2 tablespoons stevia

1   teaspoon almond extract

¾ cup stevia

¾ cup almonds, ground

Directions:

1.   In a blender, combine the avocados with the cream and the other ingredients, pulse well, divide into cups and keep in the fridge for at least 20 minutes before serving.

Nutrition: calories 106, fat 3.4, fiber 0, carbs 2.4, protein 4

Mint Rice Pudding

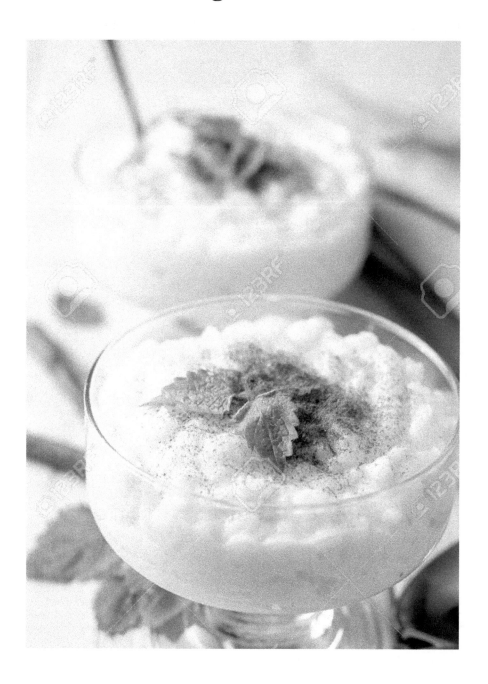

Preparation time: 10 minutes Cooking time: 30 minutes Servings: 4

Ingredients:

¼ cup stevia

2   cups cauliflower rice

2 cups coconut milk

2 tablespoons walnuts, chopped

1 tablespoon mint, chopped

1   teaspoon lime zest, grated

½ cup coconut cream

Directions:

1.   In a pan, combine the cauliflower rice with the stevia, the coconut milk and the other ingredients, whisk, bring to a simmer and cook over medium-low heat for 30 minutes.

2.   Divide the pudding into bowls and serve.

Nutrition: calories 200, fat 6.3, fiber 2, carbs 6.5, protein 8

Walnuts and Coconut Cake

Preparation time: 10 minutes Cooking time: 30 minutes Servings: 8

Ingredients:

2   cups almond flour

2 teaspoons baking powder

1 cup avocado oil

1 cup coconut flesh, unsweetened and shredded

2 cups coconut milk

1 cup stevia

1   cup coconut cream

2   tablespoons walnuts, chopped

1 tablespoon lime juice

2 teaspoons vanilla extract

Cooking spray

Directions:

1.   In a bowl, mix the almond flour with the avocado oil, the coconut flesh, coconut milk and the other ingredients except the cooking spray and whisk well.

2.   Pour the mix into a cake pan greased with the cooking spray, introduce in the oven and bake at 370 degrees F for 30 minutes.

3.   Leave the cake to cool down, cut and serve!

Nutrition: calories 200, fat 7.6, fiber 2.5, carbs 5.5, protein 4.5

Rhubarb and Berries Cream

Preparation time: 10 minutes Cooking time: 0 minutes Servings: 4

Ingredients:

2 cups rhubarb, chopped

1 cup stevia

1 cup blackberries

1 teaspoon vanilla extract

1 tablespoon avocado oil 1

/3 cup coconut cream

Directions:

1.   In a blender, combine the rhubarb with the stevia, the berries and the rest of the ingredients, pulse well, divide into cups and serve cold.

Nutrition: calories 200, fat 5.2, fiber 3.4, carbs 7.6, protein 2.5

Rice Pudding

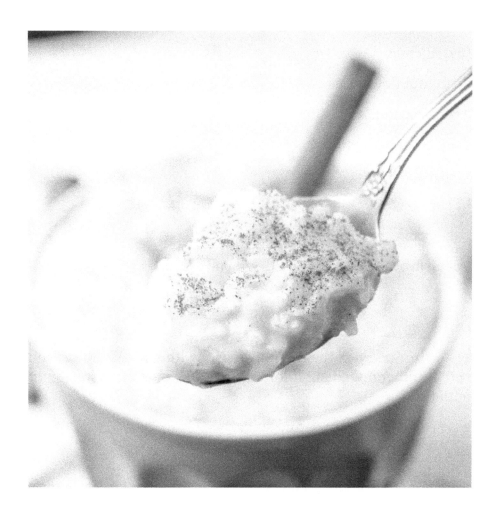

Preparation time: 10 minutes Cooking time: 20 minutes Servings: 4

Ingredients:

1 cup cauliflower rice

2 cups coconut milk

1 cup coconut cream

1 teaspoon vanilla extract

½ cup stevia

1   tablespoon cinnamon powder

½ cup avocado, peeled, pitted and cubed

Directions:

1.   In a pot, mix the cauliflower rice with the milk, the cream and the other ingredients, stir, bring to a simmer and cook for 20 minutes.

2.   Divide into bowls and serve.

Nutrition: calories 234, fat 9.5, fiber 3.4, carbs 12.4, protein 6.5

Strawberry Sorbet

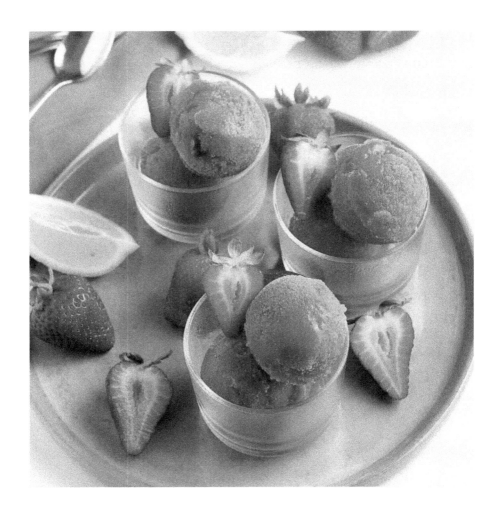

Preparation time: 3 hours Cooking time: 10 minutes Servings: 4

Ingredients:

2   cups coconut water

1 cup stevia

1 teaspoon vanilla extract

1 teaspoon lime zest, grated

1 pound strawberries, halved

Directions:

1.   Heat up a pan with the coconut water over medium heat, add berries, stevia and the other ingredients, whisk, simmer for 10 minutes, transfer to a blender, pulse, divide into bowls and keep in the freezer for 3 hours before serving.

Nutrition: calories 182, fat 5.4, fiber 3.4, carbs 12, protein 5.4

Cranberries and Avocado Pie

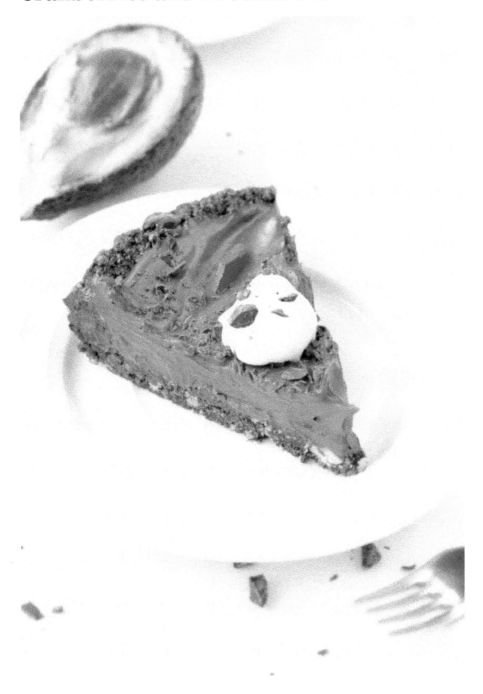

Preparation time: 10 minutes Cooking time: 40 minutes Servings: 4

Ingredients:

1 cup cranberries

1 cup avocado, peeled, pitted and mashed

1 cup coconut cream

1 cup stevia

Cooking spray

1/3 cup almond flour

1   cup coconut, unsweetened and shredded

¼ cup avocado oil

Directions:

1.   In a bowl, mix the cranberries with the avocado, the cream and the other ingredients except the cooking spray and whisk well.

2.   Grease a cake pan with the cooking spray, pour the pie mix inside and bake at 350 degrees F for 40 minutes.

3.   Cool the pie down, slice and serve.

Nutrition: calories 172, fat 3.4, fiber 4.3, carbs 11.5, protein 4.5

Lightning Source UK Ltd.
Milton Keynes UK
UKHW021845040521
383144UK00003B/367